BEAUTY: BEAUTIFUL INSIDE OUT: INNER BEAUTY
(Makeup Guide, Tips and Advice for All Ages)

By Celine War

THANK YOU!

INTRODUCTION

Thank you for downloading this book,"***Beauty: Beautiful Inside and Out: Inner Beauty, (Makeup Guide, Tips and Advice for All Ages)***".

A lot of beauty makeover books and TV shows and media we have nowadays. Most of them focused on how to improve their outward appearance so society will accept them, to boost their self-confidence, or to attract opposite sex. And there is nothing wrong with that. Surely, women really need tips and advice on how to improve ourselves—by taking care of our outward looks.

Try to consider this: Inner beauty outlasts outer beauty. And so inner beauty is what we should also enhance. There are a lot of people considered as a beauty icon not only for their external beauty, but also because of their heart for the poor, the needy, and the desolate. I have seen it on their charitable endeavors—and the beauty of their hearts far outlasts any physical beauty.

This book will share us the different tips and advice on how to improve one's beauty. And I have no doubt that this book is going to help you on your journey to discover the beauty within you!

Table of Contents

ENHANCE YOUR BEAUTY

What really is beauty? Is beauty defined by age, gender, color, body shape, or size? Or by personality, intelligence, or elegance? After all, it is hard to pinpoint the exact meaning of beauty because it really depends on the eyes of the person looking. What may seem beautiful to one person may not be to another. Just as there are no hard and fast rules when it comes to appreciating art, and there is no strict rules when it comes to appreciating a person's beauty.

In our society, the only important is to look beautiful or how to look beautiful only. Many women believe that beauty gives them an edge in getting a better job, the attention of the people around them, a handsome boyfriend, or a rich husband. Also, a lot of women believed that their status will rank high if they win a beauty pageant, become a ramp or commercial model, or work as a flight attendant. Physical beauty gives a woman confidence; it makes her feel secure. It is what the heart of every woman desires. No wonder that so many women invest a lot of money in beauty products – even if the makeup is very expensive they will buy it because they just feel it adds up in their self-esteem. Other women also feel like they look like Hollywood stars if they will buy the products endorse by them.

I am an artist, and I appreciate beauty. I admire the beautiful faces and sexy bodies of the commercial models and movie stars that I see on billboards and in TV ads. When I see them, I hope that I, too, can make myself look as pretty, sexy, and elegant. I myself have always had the dream that, one day, I can also be on TV or in magazine ads. It is awkward to say, when I was on my teen years, I only like to be a model. The problem is that I have so many moles on my face, and also I am not tall enough, and I also feel I don't look like one.

Eventually, through the years, I got interested on makeup. I enrolled for a make-up course so that I could enhance my features, and so that I could also earn extra as a part-time make-up artist. I bought a lot of makeup! On my mind, I will get the amount I invested by working myself as a make-up artist. At that time, I replace all of the points I got on my credit card for gift certificates at Rustan's to buy a makeup. I gathered together a big, varied collection of high-quality eye shadow sets, lipsticks, blush, foundation, BB creams, and pressed powders. I also accumulated quality mascara, eyeliner, brushes, tweezers, and lash curlers. But sadly, I was not able to use all of them. Others have expired. And after many years of putting on makeup on family members and friends, I have not earned a single cent.

This is one reason why I thought of writing a book that will give you, dear reader, and practical tips on how to enhance your physical beauty. This book gives ideas on how to define your features with makeup. To some degree, makeup can help emphasize your best features. You won't need a formal make-up lesson – all you need is basic make-up products and tools, and you have to practice. In this book, I have included a list of the basic make-up products and tools that you will need. You will be encouraged to see how makeup can enhance your looks and how it can increase your confidence.

In a bigger picture, how important makeup really is to a woman? The most important question may – is this the only way we can be truly attractive, truly beautiful? How about if you can't afford to buy a makeup? Bottom line, we women must realize that we do not have to invest so much money in beauty products in order to look beautiful. There is more important than physical beauty. The Bible tells us that being beautiful is not about looks.

We learn that beauty does not come from outward adornment, clothes, jewelry, hair, or makeup. There is something more to being beautiful on the outside, something that, in the eyes of everyone, is even more valuable. This is our inner beauty. This is the beauty that won't fade away, even as we age. Think about this – do you have a friend which is not that pretty looking but you like to spend time with her a lot? Why? Because she has a unique features. This is called inner beauty. In such a woman, we can see in her eyes and in the she speaks that she has a good heart. Her aura is radiant, and the sincerity of her heart and her kindness cannot be ignored. She is nice to talk with. She is easy to get along with. She is always happy. Nobody talks bad stuffs to her. All the words that came from her mouth are positive and give compliment. What comes out of our mouth reveals what is in our heart.

If you are finding tips on how to be beautiful, this book is right just for you. As you read, you will learn not just how to put on makeup, but also what it means to be beautiful inside. Makeup is just a small part of this book, and it is not the important part. This book is about having inner beauty, the beauty that truly lasts. May this book be a guide to enhancing your outer and inner beauty.

WHY DO WOMEN WEAR MAKEUP?

A lot of people told me that I am not easy to get along with. In my younger years, I was not the kind of person that you would have liked to have for a friend. My sister once said, "I couldn't get along with you before because you were different." And I thought that it was so kind of her to put it that way because honestly, she meant "difficult" maybe. Maybe my facial features are the one intimidating to people. I have Chinese ancestors and a Spanish great-grandmother, mestiza in features. Way back I thought that being mestiza is an asset of mine, but then it was a hindrance for me to have a relationship because the first guys would thought of me is a monster.

My growing-up years had an impact on my later years as an adult. I feel like I was superior over those who were not like me. I easily felt irritated, for instance, with people who were slow to understand simple instructions. I also had a little need for friends, and I liked taking charge and being in control of situations. I would get into conflicts with my sisters, classmates, clients, business partners, in-laws, household helpers, and drivers. But by God's grace, He opened my eyes to see my own flaws and through various circumstances, He humbled me.

In our society, being beautiful is an asset. But from my story, we will see that there is more to beauty than just the physical. It is really the kind of character you have that will determine whether or not you are beautiful.

Even so, it is all right to take care of our physical beauty. And knowing how to put on makeup properly is one way of doing this. Taking care of our outer beauty -- this is just one thing for us to reason out why girls wear makeup. Let's look into the other reasons why.

To be attractive to the opposite sex

When I asked some women why they wear makeup, this is what they said:

"Of course, I want to be beautiful! To have more suitors."

"I want to look beautiful so that my husband will not exchange me for a younger woman."

"I like it when men look at me."

"I am getting old and I'm still single. I need to be beautiful."

"I like to be beautiful when my boyfriend is around."

Some ladies think that a lot of makeup will make them look sophisticated and will therefore make them look more attractive to men. But I also know that many men do not like makeup on their partners. There are a lot of guys who like their partners look simple – and it doesn't mean that their partners don't need to dress up for their man.

It is essential to put on makeup so that we can look beautiful in the eyes of our spouse or boyfriend, but we don't have to be obsessed. Our makeup should match our personality. It should also go with the occasion and the place we are visiting. You can also ask your partner on what they would wear so that you could match your outfit with his. If your partner will take you out on a date, ask him where you will go. If he says he will take you to a movie, you can have a daytime or sporty make-up look. Maybe your partner would feel insecure if you put on a lot of makeup and he would look like your bodyguard instead.

To feel good about ourselves

For many women, putting on makeup and going to a hair salon simply means that they just want to feel good, look good, and be pretty. (There is something about the parlor that lures women to go and be pampered. In my younger years, we called this as a parlor. Going to salons may be relaxing and I don't see anything wrong with them. But does it really make us relax or relieve your stress when we go there? It could be make you relax or relieve your stress for a short time but when it comes in real life, we may still need to face a difficult husband, unruly kids, disobedient helpers, financial difficulties, and various household problems.

We can't get away from our everyday problems. But when the stresses of life come, putting on makeup is a simple way to feel good about ourselves. It is a small thing, but looking good and being well-groomed can help us feel better! Even at the office, and you have to deal with an unreasonable boss, and piles of work – looking good will not solve these problems. But knowing that you look good can help you feel good and feel more in control.

The next time you go to a party and you don't have confidence of what you wear, you can focus on carefully putting on your makeup. Even if you are only wearing a simple dress or a T-shirt, carefully applied makeup can boost your confidence and help you feel good about yourself. If you put on your makeup really good, this can also help you overcome your insecurities.

To cover blemishes and skin discolorations

"I have a dark scar on my forehead."

"A lot of hyperpigmentation spots that is why I use BB cream."

"I am getting old. I really need to hide the lines on my eyes."

A lot of women can't get out of the house when they were not wearing makeup, and even not wearing lipstick. I, for one, do not like to go out of the house unless I have on at least some eyeliner, lipstick, and BB cream. When I am talking to someone, it gives me confidence when I know that I have makeup on.

When women wear makeup, it makes them look presentable and well-groomed. Good makeup can cover the imperfections on our face. If we have scars and hyperpigmentation spots, these can make our facial skin look uneven and discolored. This is why we need to learn how to cover them with good makeup.

The ageing process can affect our facial features. A woman who enters the age of forty can begin to feel that she is ageing. Women started to worry about the wrinkles and dark circles under her eyes. When the hyperpigmentation spots on her face increase, she begins to panic. This is actually one of the reasons why makeup was invented – it can really help improve our looks and make us more attractive. A good BB cream or CC cream does a great job in covering our flaws, and it also works as a moisturizer, sunblock, and for some brands, as a skin whitener.

To define and accentuate facial features

"Everyone wants to look beautiful. I put on makeup to enhance my eyes. My eyes are my asst."

"My cheekbones look beautiful, so I emphasize them with blush."

"I don't have an eyebrow, that's why I can't go out of the house without shading my brow area with an eyebrow pencil."

Every woman has unique facial features that make her special and beautiful in her own way. It's our assets, and makeup does a lot to define and accentuate these assets. Example, some women got insecure of having a full lip. But the truth is, full lips are an asset – think of Angelina Jolie! So if you have full lips you should emphasize these – wear lipstick!

We can use makeup to draw attention away from features we may not be comfortable with. Example, if your eyes are already beautiful but you are not happy with having a low nasal bridge; you can use makeup to fully emphasize your eyes. On the other hand, if you have nicely shaped lips but you have pimples on your cheeks, you can highlight your lips with a good lip liner and lipstick. Doing so will draw people's attention away from your pimples.

HOW DO WOMEN PUT ON THEIR MAKEUP?

Makeup gives every woman the power to look great and have different personas. If you like to look beautiful, you need to bring out the creativity in you. Try the different styles and products so you can get your desired image that you have projected. So we can maximize the impact that makeup gives, we need to have the correct make-up products and tools.

Here are the basic make-up products that women must have,

Foundation

It will make your skin tone fair and so, your face will look smoother. It will also cover the hyperpigmentation spots and discoloration.

Types of foundation:

- Liquid
- Stick
- Cream to powder
- Powder compact
- BB cream – this is a great product that covers your hyperpigmentation spots. I personally recommend Korean brands since they were developed for Korean women, whose skin tone is similar to us.

  - Choose a foundation shade that matches your skin tone.
  - Apply and blend foundation with a foundation brush or a latex sponge. You may also use your fingers.
  - Spread foundation evenly on your face, starting from the hairline. Apply also on your neck.
  - Avoid applying a thick foundation so your face won't look artificial

- If you have an oily face, apply astringent first before you put on foundation. It's good to use powder compact if you have an oily face.
- If you have a dry skin, use liquid foundation.

Concealer

Cover ups your dark blemishes and scars, and also you under-eye dark circles, discoloration, and redness.

Types of concealer:

- Liquid
- Stick
    - Use concealer which matches your skin tone.
    - Apply concealer by using a flathead brush with synthetic bristles. You may also use your fingers.
    - Apply concealer only on areas that need to be covered, such as hyperpigmentation spots, under-eye dark circles, and scars.
    - Use a little amount when applying.

Powder

It is important to put on powder, so the foundation and concealer won't lock-in, and to get rid of a shiny face.

Types of powder:

- Pressed powder
- Loose powder
  - Apply powder with a powder brush or powder puff.
  - Sometimes 2-in-1 pressed powder also used as a foundation on daily use.
  - Beauty sections in department stores, you can find different brands of 2-in-1 pressed powder. You can also apply it dry or wet.
  - Make sure powder puff is always clean. Accumulated dirt can give rise to bacteria and can harm your skin.

Blush

With the right blush, a natural flush and glow are restored to your skin.

Types of blush:

- Powder (the most commonly used)
- Cream (have natural effect)
- Liquid or gel
  - When buying liquid or gel blush, choose the type which matches your skin -- whether normal, oily, or dry.
  - If you use cream blush, or liquid or gel, you may use a contour cream brush for application; you may also use your fingers.
  - Apply blush on your cheeks. To emphasize your cheekbones, use a darker shade of blush under each cheekbone. In daytime, use a lighter shade of blush on the apples of your cheeks. In nighttime, apply darker shade. Blend well.
  - Coordinate the color of your blush with the color of your lipstick. Make sure that it matches with the one you are wearing.

Eyebrow Makeup

Our eyebrows need to be properly filled in and shaped well.

Types of eyebrow makeup:

- Pencil (most popular)
- Powder
- Cream
  - Brush your eyebrows first before you shape it.
  - Shape your brows with an eyebrow pencil. Using tweezers, pluck the hair that is not within the line you have drawn.
  - Your eyebrow hair can no longer grow if you always get it, so be careful. There are different techniques for shaping your brows – like threading, that salon practices, or shaving, or simply plucking with tweezers.
  - If you have a short eyebrow, you can use an eyebrow pencil to extend your brows a little, over the tip of your eyes.
  - Use taupe, charcoal or dark brown color.

Using the right eye shadow enhances our eyes. Our eyes can really stand out.

Types of eye shadow:

- Powder (most popular)
- Cream (good for dry skin)
- Pencil (easy to use)
    - If you are a contact-lens wearer, be extra careful while working on your eyes.
    - Apply eye shadow on your eyelids with a flathead or full head shadow brush.
    - Eye-shadow brushes that are dome-shaped are the best to use.
    - Carefully blend your eye shadow for a clean, seamless look.
    - There is a wide variety of eye-shadow colors to choose from. A lot of these eye shadows have matte or metallic finish.
    - If it is daytime, use a lighter shade of eye shadow. Darker shade, or smokey-eye effect, for evening.

Eyeliner

The eyeliner defines and enhances our eyes.

Types of eyeliner:

- Pencil
- Kohl
- Powder
- Gel
- Cream
    - The most convenient eyeliner to use is the pencil. But the cream eyeliner also works well since it is easy to apply, when you use a fine-point eyeliner brush.
    - Start lining from the outer corner of you eye.
    - When doing the lower eye area, gently pull down on the skin below your eyelid. Draw a line close to the lashes.
    - Use brown shade in daytime and black shade in nighttime.

Mascara

Good mascara enhances and draws attention to our eyes. It also makes our eyelashes look longer and thicker.

Types of mascara:

- Lengthening
- Thickening
- Curling
  - All mascaras come with a brush and are easy to apply.
  - Curl your eyelashes first before applying mascara. Use eyelash curler.
  - Sweep the mascara brush from side to side, and then brush outward. You can also use eyelash grooming brush to separate the lashes evenly.
  - Use brown shade during daytime and black shade during nighttime.
  - Mascara has a short shelf life. In six months, your mascara will dry up, and you will need to get a new one.

Lip Color

Lip color enhances our lips and adds color to them.

Types of lip color:

- Sheer lipstick (have a little pigment)
- Shimmery lipstick (metallic or pearly)
- Cream lipstick (have emollients)
- Lip stain (can dry lips)
- Long-wearing lipstick (this can look dry)
  - Lip color can be applied directly or by using a lip brush.
  - First, line your lips with a lip pencil. Fill the entire area of the lips.
  - If your eye shadow is dark, it is best to use a light color for your lips, and vice versa.
  - Use bolder lip color for evening.

Here are the tools you will need,

- Latex sponge (disposable) – for applying liquid foundation
- Powder puff -- for application of pressed powder
- Powder brush – for application of loose powder
- Blusher brush – for application of blush
- Contour cream brush – for application of blush
- Flathead brush – dome-shaped, with synthetic bristles, for applying eye shadow or concealer
- Eye shadow brush – dome-shaped
- Eyeliner brush – with a fine, pointy tip
- Angled liner brush – with soft and firm bristles
- Lip brush – with small, flat and firm bristles
- Eyelash grooming brush
- Eyelash curler
- Tweezers – for plucking and shaping eyebrows

Steps in applying makeup,

- Wash your face with a facial soap or cleanser, choose the product that matches your skin whether oily, normal, or dry.
- Apply moisturizer and let it set for five minutes before you apply makeup.
- Apply foundation or BB cream in your face, starting from the hairline and down to the chin. Also apply in the neck.
- Apply concealer, if needed.
- Shape your eyebrows.
- Apply eye shadow.
- Apply eyeliner.
- Apply mascara.
- Apply blush.
- Apply loose powder or pressed powder.
- Shape your lips with a lip liner.
- Apply lipstick.
- Apply lip gloss so your lips won't be dry.

THE FIVE BASIC MAKE-UP LOOKS

The Sporty Look

If your personality is laid-back type and you like sports, this is the look that best fits you. When you go out on a casual setting

To clubhouse, sports arena, or mall, sporty look is the right one for you.

- Foundation
- Concealer (only if needed)
- Powder (matte)
- Blush
- Fill in eyebrows
- Mascara (curl lashes first before applying)
- Lipstick (sheen or gloss)

The Daytime Look

If you are going to church, a lunch party, or a lunch date with your spouse or boyfriend, this look will be perfect for you.

- Foundation
- Concealer (only if needed)
- Powder
- Blush
- Fill in eyebrows
- Eye shadow (brownish shade for eyelid)
- Mascara
- Lipstick

The Corporate Look

For all the women who work on a corporate world, for business executives, managers, supervisors, and others who work in an office, this is the look right for you.

- Foundation
- Concealer (only if needed)
- Powder
- Blush (natural shade; consider the color amber)
- Fill in eyebrows
- Eye shadow – highlight as needed
- Eyeliner – line upper lids with brown or dark brown liner
- Mascara (dark brown or black)
- Lip color – use a shade slightly darker than the natural color of your lips

The Elegant Look

If you attend a wedding, or night party, this looks is best fits you.

- Foundation
- Concealer
- Powder (slight sheen)
- Blush
- Fill in eyebrows
- Eye contour – highlight, shadow as needed
- Eye shadow
- Eyeliner – for the upper lid, dark brown, gray or black color
- Mascara
- Lip color – coordinate with the color of your eye shadow. If your shadow is light, you may use a darker lip color.

The Sexy Look

You must know how to carry this type of look! This doesn't mean that you have to wear sexy clothes or expose your skin to look sexy. Most of the time, sexiness stems from confidence – the "it" factor.

- Foundation
- Concealer
- Powder (slight sheen)
- Blush – coordinate with lip color
- Fill in eyebrows
- Eye shadow
- Eyeliner – highlight, shade as needed with dark brown, gray or black eyeliner; increase thickness of liner
- Mascara – you may want to try false eyelashes
- Lip color

YOUR SELF-WORTH

In God's eyes, every woman has worth. The sad thing is, often, we base our self-worth not on His love for us, but on the wrong things – and this includes how people see us.

We base our self-worth on our looks

A beautiful face can certainly elevate our self-esteem. But once a woman has been labeled "ugly", or "short", it will have a negative impact on the way she sees herself and relates with others.

There was a time when Nick Vujicic, the man born without arms and legs, also believed in a lie. He believed that he could never fend for himself, get a job, get married or have children. Because of what he looks, people made fun of him. But Nick's parents loved him, and they introduced him to Jesus Christ. When he started reading the Bible, he then realized how much God loves him and how beautiful he already is in His eyes. Nick's message and core of his worldwide ministry – God loves us, and we are all beautiful, for we were created in His own image.

We base our self-worth on our accomplishments

In this competitive world, many people base their self-worth on accomplishments, position, and titles. In corporate world, we can already hear many stories about people who would do anything to get to a higher position. Because they believed that status and achievements are everything.

The feeling of being able to accomplish something of your own and to have the power to buy your wants and needs is really a good feeling. Being able to do great things or being able to reach our goals can make us happy, but it this happiness won't last long. On the other hand, when we give our time and attention to the truly important things in life, we will receive joy that lasts. Blessings will pour upon us, a blessing so great that these cannot even be compared to any earthly achievement.

For us women, we need to remember that being beautiful and having high-status job will never complete us. It won't last. One day, our beauty will fade. And while our career may be good while we are young, one day, we will also need to retire. We cannot base our self-worth on these temporary things.

We base our self-worth on our possessions

Many women use money to try to raise their self-worth. If we have enough savings or acquire extra money, we think that we now have the ability to "make ourselves more important." A lot of us women bought expensive products which previously we can't afford. Buy beauty products, expensive bags and shoes, jewelry and watches, and expensive clothing. We feel good when we have these things.

Do these possessions really change our self-worth? only temporarily. I know certain women who have everything, and yet, they are not happy. Something is missing in their lives. Going to a party, looking so elegant with their beautiful jewelry and clothes. They seem happy but when you look into their eyes, they are not. They are materialistic and discontented.

Acquiring wealth is exciting, but it comes with great responsibility. God blesses us with gifts not for us to boast, but so that we can use them properly.

Some words about our self-worth and ageing

If we are honest with ourselves, we will admit that a lot of times we are hesitant to disclose our real age. For many women, ageing have effects on their self-esteem.

Beauty is not synonymous to youth! We should always remember that we have to act our age. Let's show the wisdom we have accumulated over the years.

Ageing is Inevitable. Fighting it will cost a lot of money and will lead only to frustration. Outer beauty is temporary. When we spend too much time beautifying ourselves, it will lead to self-centeredness, our ego will be feed, and we will miss out on God's plan for us at this stage in our life.

WHAT MAKES A WOMAN UGLY?

We can say that being evil makes a person look ugly. Sin makes us look ugly – both in the eyes of other people and in the eyes of God. It is what's stored inside our hearts that will reveal our true character.

Envy, Jealousy

An envious and jealous woman craves and covets someone or something that belongs to another. She will not be contented nor thankful. She has resentment because she desires the advantages, possessions, or attainments that another may have. She always gets jealous to other people. What people have, she also want it.

Self-Centeredness

The conceited and self-centered woman is focused on herself and on her own interests. She builds up her own image while tearing down that of others. She talks about herself all the time. She is insensitive about others need. She is selfish with her time, knowledge, and thoughts. She don't care for others – has her own world.

The opposite of conceit and self-centeredness is compassion for others.

Malice

The malicious woman desires to inflict pain or suffering on another by deliberately lying. She has hatred. And she really wants to harm another person. Tells false statement about others and think harmful thoughts to others.

There is no direct opposite of malice, but if we truly love and always seek the good of others, we will not be malicious.

Being a Gossip

They bring judgment on themselves. They get into the habit of being idle. And not only do they become idlers, but also gossips and busybodies. The gossiper reveals the secrets of others. She maliciously talks about someone to another person who has no business knowing about what is being said. Gossipers only intention is to build up herself only and she does this by making other people bad. Exposing others failures to others.

The opposite of being a gossiper is being someone who cares enough about other to respect their reputation and privacy.

Being a Slanderer

The woman who slanders is a woman who maliciously gives false statements about others.

The opposite of being a slanderer is being someone who does not spread lies about others.

Materialism

The materialistic woman is fascinated with acquiring and caring for things like expensive clothing, shoes, bags, and jewelry. She likes to flaunt her things in front of other people, and she talks about them all the time. She only work and save only to buy different kind of luxury items. She always find things that makes her happy. She feels that having a Chanel or a Louis Vuitton bag could add beauty.

The opposite of materialism is also simplicity and contentment.

Being Judgmental

The judgmental woman likes to assume, and she has a conclusion about every person and situation. She magnifies the faults of other people, while excusing her own weakness. In order to build herself up, she criticized others. She always feels that she's always right.

The opposite of being judgmental is being someone who is tolerant and broad-minded.

Bitterness, Unforgiving

For this woman, she never let go of her past. Always reminding about how she got hurt by the ones they love. Even in her sleep, she could dream about getting revenge to those who have offended her. She harbors an intense hostility towards another person. This woman is cynical, cold, harsh, and refuses to forgive and to forget. She allows bitterness to rule over her heart, and she is not open to reconciliation.

The opposite of being unforgiving and bitter is being someone who is forgiving and who does not harbor grudges.

WHAT MAKES A WOMAN BEAUTIFUL?

Your beauty should not come from outward adornment, such as braided hair and the wearing of gold jewelry and fine clothes. Instead it should be that of you inner self, the unfading beauty of a gentle and quiet spirit, which is of great worth in God's sight.

In our world today, we are consumed by our selfish desires and ambitions, so much so that we miss out on the greater and more important things in life. I am not perfect; but in all humility, I can say that I am no longer the woman that I was before. Patience, kindness, gentleness, simplicity, unconditional love, and perseverance are the characteristics of a true beauty have.

Love

Love is not a feeling; it is a gift given by God. No amount of work or money can make us love the way God wants us to love.

Joy

Joy is what we will feel deep in our hearts.

Peace

Peace is the result of having a deep relation with God.

Patience

Patience is being able to withstand trials and endure pain without complaining.

Kindness, Goodness, Gentleness

When we have these in our life, we are tender, benevolent, and helpful to others. Everything we do is acted upon by grace. A kind person shows concern for others, speaks gently, and is not easily angered.

Faithfulness

Being faithful means being reliable and steadfast. Faithfulness is a key factor on a relationship.

Self-Control

Self-control is the ability to rein in and manage one's self. It is the strength and ability to say "No to temptation and to sin. Many women struggle with controlling themselves in the areas of gossiping, excessive shopping, and nagging.

CONCLUSION

Once again, I give my greats THANKS TO YOU for downloading my book.

I hope that this book *Beauty: Beautiful Inside and Out: Inner Beauty, (Makeup Guide, Tips and Advice for All Ages)"* has taught you not only the basic makeover, but also what really beauty is within you.

I have tried to keep things simple as it should be.

I hope that, now you have more knowledge on how to enhance your beauty you will continue with your learning and go on to a more advanced program. Remember that being beautiful inside and out is the most important in beauty.

Thank you for downloading my book; if this book helped you in any way, I'd like to ask you for a favor to be kind and leave a review for this book on Amazon. Your feedback will help me create more quality content that will help you!

Thanks,

Celine War